CHELATION THERAPY

A Comprehensive Guide to
Cardiovascular Health, and Chronic
Disease Management Through Targeted
Heavy Metal Detoxification

By

Sharon G. Brown

Copyright @2024

TABLE OF CONTENT

CHAPTER ONE 8

Introduction to Chelation Therapy 8

   Causes of Heavy Metal Exposure 14

   Effects of Heavy Metal Accumulation on Health 17

CHAPTER TWO 20

   Symptoms of Heavy Metal Poisoning 20

   Medical Assessment or Diagnosis 22

   Chelation Agents and Methods 24

   Synthetic Chelators 31

CHAPTER THREE 34

   Natural Chelators 34

   Herbal Chelation Remedies 43

   Protocols for Chelation Therapy 47

CHAPTER FOUR 52

Oral Chelation Therapy 52

Methods of Chelation Administration....55

Applications and Benefits of Chelation Therapy..62

CHAPTER FIVE 98

Diet, Lifestyle, and Chelation 98

Lifestyle Practices to Improve Effective Chelation 100

Ensuring Safety and Managing Risk......104

Advancements in Chelation Delivery Methods..111

Integrating Chelation with Other Therapies...113

END 116

Revolutionizing Health through Heavy Metal Removal

Imagine a treatment that can rid your body of dangerous heavy metals, enhance heart health, and even provide relief for chronic ailments. This is not science fiction; it is the promise of chelation therapy, a medical procedure based on detoxification and rejuvenation.

Chelation therapy involves administering chelating agents, which are chemicals that bind to heavy metals and minerals in the body allowing them to be eliminated. Chelation therapy, which was first created to treat heavy metal poisoning, has now evolved to treat a wide range of health concerns, such as atherosclerosis, neurological illnesses (Autism spectrum disorders, brain tumors, cerebral palsy and ADD,), and cardiovascular disease.

This guide will provide you with the following:

- A thorough examination of the history, mechanisms of chelation therapy
- Several approaches to chelation, such as EDTA, DMSA and natural chelators.
- Detailed protocols that demonstrate the practical implementation of chelation therapy.
- Potential advantages, hazards, and the most recent scientific discoveries that substantiate the effectiveness of chelation therapy.

- The significance of tailored treatment regimens and the influence of diet and lifestyle in optimizing the advantages of detoxification.

Whether you are a healthcare practitioner, a patient seeking alternative treatments, or simply inquisitive about the latest medical developments, this book offers useful insights and practical guidance on incorporating chelation therapy into a comprehensive health plan. Acquire the necessary knowledge to make well-informed decisions regarding your health and explore the potential of obtaining optimal well-being via the strategic application of chelation therapy.

CHAPTER ONE

Introduction to Chelation Therapy

Chelation therapy is a medical procedure employed to eliminate heavy metals and other toxic substances from the body. The term "chelation" is derived from the Greek word "chele," which means "claw." This phrase is used to describe the process by which chelating agents attach to heavy metals, creating a complex that can be eliminated from the body.

This therapy is predominantly recognized for its application in the treatment of heavy metal intoxication, including lead or mercury toxicity. The process entails the introduction of chelating agents that travel in the bloodstream, attaching to heavy metals and aiding in their elimination through urine.

Chelation treatment has its roots in the early 20th century and was first created during World War II as a means to treat lead poisoning in individuals who were exposed to lead in battery manufacturing and munitions industries. Ethylenediaminetetraacetic acid (EDTA), the initial man-made chelating agent, was produced during the 1930s. EDTA chelation therapy garnered considerable interest in the 1950s for its application in treating heavy metal intoxication and subsequently for cardiovascular ailments, owing to its capacity to sequester calcium in arterial plaque.

Throughout the years, the utilization of chelation therapy has extended beyond the treatment of immediate cases of severe heavy metal toxicity. Scientists and medical professionals investigated the possible applications of this treatment for long-term health concerns such as atherosclerosis, neurological illnesses, and autistic spectrum disorders. Despite the disagreement and doubt among medical professionals, ongoing scientific investigation and feedback from patients have consistently backed the investigation of chelation therapy as a supplementary form of treatment.

Chelation therapy functions based on the theory of chemical bonding. The chelating compounds employed in this treatment have a high attraction towards heavy metals and minerals, resulting in the formation of stable complexes that can be readily eliminated from the body.

Some examples of key chelating agents are:

- EDTA, also known as Ethylenediaminetetraacetic Acid, is a commonly used substance for the treatment of lead poisoning and cardiovascular disorders. It works by binding to calcium and lead, which helps in their elimination from the body.

- DMSA (Dimercaptosuccinic Acid) is an oral chelator that is highly efficient in treating lead, mercury, and arsenic poisoning, especially in juvenile patients.

- DMPS (Dimercaptopropane-1-sulfonate) is an oral chelator that is frequently chosen for the purpose of mercury detoxification.
- Alpha-lipoic acid, cilantro, and chlorella are natural chelators that have become increasingly popular due to their milder detoxifying properties. These agents augment the body's innate detoxification processes and are frequently incorporated into comprehensive health plans.

The efficiency of chelation therapy relies on several aspects, such as the kind and extent of heavy metal exposure, the selection of the chelating agent, and the specific health conditions of the patient.

Conducting comprehensive assessments and creating individualized treatment plans are essential for maximizing benefits and minimizing potential hazards.

Chelation therapy is a flexible and developing treatment method with a significant past and a strong scientific basis. The use of this method is extensive, ranging from treating acute poisoning to managing chronic health concerns. It provides hope and healing by carefully eliminating poisonous heavy metals from the body.

Causes of Heavy Metal Exposure

Heavy metals are naturally existing chemical components that possess the potential to be harmful to the body, even when present in small amounts. Typical sources of heavy metal exposure encompass:

- Environmental Pollution: Environmental pollution is caused by industrial activities, such as mining, smelting, and manufacturing, which result in the discharge of heavy metals into the air, water, and soil. Lead and mercury are frequently present in industrial pollutants, as an illustration.

- Contaminated Water: Drinking water may be tainted with heavy metals such as lead, arsenic, and cadmium due to the presence of natural mineral deposits, industrial discharges, and agricultural runoff.

- Food Sources: Heavy metals have the ability to build up in the food chain. Both fish and shellfish may contain elevated levels of mercury. Lead, cadmium, and arsenic can be found in fruits and vegetables that are cultivated in soil or water that is contaminated.

- Household Products: Numerous household commodities, including batteries, paints, plumbing supplies, and cosmetics, can serve as reservoirs of heavy metals such as lead, mercury, and cadmium.

- Occupational Exposure: Individuals employed in sectors such as mining, welding, construction, and battery manufacture face an elevated likelihood of being exposed to heavy metals.

- Traditional Medicines and Supplements: Certain traditional remedies and herbal supplements may include substantial amounts of heavy metals, especially if obtained from polluted areas.

Effects of Heavy Metal Accumulation on Health

Heavy metal accumulation in the body can result in many health problems, impacting multiple organ systems. Primary health effects encompass:

- **Neurological Effects:** Heavy metals such as lead and mercury have neurotoxic properties and can result in cognitive impairments, memory decline, emotional disturbances, and developmental delays in children. Prolonged exposure can result in the development of neurodegenerative disorders, such as Alzheimer's and Parkinson's diseases.

- **Cardiovascular Issues:** Heavy metals have the potential to harm blood vessels, elevate blood pressure, and contribute to the progression of atherosclerosis, ultimately resulting in heart attacks and strokes.

- **Renal Damage:** Heavy metal intoxication can cause significant harm to the kidneys, resulting in reduced kidney function, chronic renal disease, and, in severe cases, kidney failure.

- **Reproductive Health:** The presence of heavy metals can have detrimental effects on reproductive health, leading to infertility, miscarriages, and developmental problems in fetuses.

- **Immunosuppression:** Heavy metals have the ability to impair the immune system, making it more vulnerable to infections and autoimmune disorders.

- **Carcinogenic Effects:** Certain heavy metals, such as arsenic and cadmium, are categorized as carcinogens and have been associated with the development of different types of cancer, including lung, bladder, and skin cancer.

CHAPTER TWO

Symptoms of Heavy Metal Poisoning

The symptoms of heavy metal toxicity might differ based on the specific type and extent of exposure. Typical indications comprise:

Lead Poisoning:

Symptoms of lead poisoning include abdominal pain, constipation, exhaustion, headaches, irritability, memory issues, and in severe cases, seizures.

Mercury Poisoning:

Symptoms of mercury poisoning include tremors, anxiety, irritability, cognitive impairment, abnormalities in vision and hearing, and muscle weakness.

Arsenic Poisoning:

Arsenic poisoning is characterized by dermatological alterations such as skin darkening or thickness, as well as gastrointestinal symptoms including nausea, vomiting, diarrhea, and stomach pain. In chronic situations, it can lead to the development of skin lesions and even cancer.

Cadmium Poisoning:

Cadmium Poisoning can lead to respiratory problems, kidney impairment, bone discomfort, and fractures.

Medical Assessment or Diagnosis

The process of diagnosing heavy metal toxicity entails multiple steps:

1. Medical History and Physical Examination: An extensive inquiry into probable sources of exposure and a comprehensive physical examination to detect indications of toxicity.

2. Diagnostic examinations conducted in a laboratory setting:

- Blood tests are conducted to determine the concentrations of metals such as lead, mercury, and cadmium.

- Urine tests are used to evaluate the quantities of heavy metals excreted by the body.
- Hair and Nail Analysis: Assess prolonged exposure by quantifying the concentration of metals in hair and nails.
- Imaging and functional tests may be required to evaluate the severity of organ damage. For example, X-rays can be used to detect lead lines in bones, while kidney function tests can examine the functioning of the kidneys.

Prompt identification and timely action are essential in effectively managing heavy metal toxicity in order to mitigate potential long-term health ramifications. Chelation therapy is crucial for lowering the accumulation of heavy metals and alleviating the related health hazards.

Chelation Agents and Methods

EDTA is widely utilized as a chelating agent due to its effectiveness in treating lead poisoning and other heavy metal toxicities. This compound has the ability to bind to different metals, creating complexes that are stable and can dissolve in water. These complexes can then be eliminated from the body through urine. EDTA functions by forming complexes with metal ions, including lead, calcium, and iron, through binding. This binding process decreases the presence of these metals in the body, preventing the formation of harmful compounds and reducing their toxic effects. EDTA is commonly used intravenously to treat acute heavy metal poisoning. However, there are also oral and rectal forms available for less severe cases.

Applications:

• **Lead Poisoning:** EDTA has proven to be extremely effective in lowering blood lead levels and preventing neurological damage caused by lead exposure.

• **Cardiovascular Diseases:** The potential benefits of EDTA chelation therapy in treating atherosclerosis have been investigated. It has been suggested that this therapy could enhance blood flow by binding to calcium in arterial plaques. EDTA is also utilized in situations involving hypercalcemia and specific forms of iron overload.

- EDTA is commonly used for general detoxification purposes to eliminate various heavy metals, including cadmium and mercury.

Administration:

Intravenous administration is the usual method for EDTA, although there are also oral formulations available. For acute poisoning and more severe cases, intravenous administration is the preferred method.

Common side effects of this medication include mild gastrointestinal upset, fatigue, and hypocalcemia (low calcium levels). These effects can be easily managed through proper monitoring and supplementation.

DMSA (Dimercaptosuccinic Acid): DMSA is an orally administered chelating agent that is highly effective for treating heavy metal poisoning in both children and adults. This treatment has been approved by the FDA for the management of lead poisoning.

The mechanism of action involves the binding of DMSA to heavy metals such as lead, mercury, and arsenic. This binding forms a water-soluble complex that is then excreted in the urine. Its strong attraction to lead and mercury allows it to effectively lower their levels in the body.

Applications:

• **Lead Poisoning:** DMSA is commonly prescribed as the initial treatment for lead poisoning in individuals of all ages.

- **Mercury Poisoning:** It is also utilized off-label to address mercury toxicity.

• DMSA can also be used to treat heavy metal poisoning caused by **arsenic** and **cadmium**.

Administration:

DMSA is typically taken orally, usually in the form of capsules. The dosage and duration of treatment are determined by factors such as the severity of the poisoning and the patient's age and weight.

Possible side effects of this medication include gastrointestinal disturbances, skin rashes, and mild elevations in liver enzymes. When used under medical supervision, it is typically well-tolerated.

DMPS (Dimercaptopropane-1-sulfonate)

DMPS is a synthetic chelator commonly used for the purpose of mercury detoxification. This medication can be given either orally or intravenously, and it is well-known for its high level of effectiveness and safety.

The mechanism of action involves the binding of DMPS to heavy metals like mercury, arsenic, and lead. This binding forms a stable complex that is then excreted in the urine. Its strong affinity for mercury makes it a popular option for mercury detoxification.

Applications:

- **Mercury Poisoning:** DMPS is commonly utilized in the treatment of mercury toxicity, specifically in cases related to dental amalgams and environmental exposure.

• It is also effective for treating **arsenic** and **lead poisoning**.

Administration:

DMPS can be given either orally or intravenously. The administration method and dosage are determined by the severity of the poisoning and individual patient characteristics.

Side effects typically manifest as mild symptoms such as allergic reactions, gastrointestinal upset, and alterations in liver enzyme levels. Thorough medical supervision can help to minimize these risks.

Synthetic Chelators

Penicillamine:

Penicillamine is a chelating agent commonly prescribed for the treatment of Wilson's disease, a condition characterized by abnormal copper metabolism, as well as rheumatoid arthritis. Penicillamine has additional applications beyond treating Wilson's disease. It is capable of chelating heavy metals such as lead and mercury.

Serious side effects, including bone marrow suppression, kidney damage, and severe allergic reactions, may occur, leading to reduced usage for heavy metal detoxification.

Deferoxamine

Deferoxamine is a medication that is commonly prescribed to individuals with iron overload conditions like thalassemia and hemochromatosis. It works by acting as an iron-chelating agent, effectively reducing the levels of iron in the body. It is not commonly employed for general heavy metal detoxification, but it is remarkably efficient in lowering iron levels.

Some potential side effects of this medication include visual and auditory disturbances, gastrointestinal issues, and allergic reactions.

Deferiprone and Deferasirox

Deferiprone and Deferasirox are both oral iron chelators that are commonly prescribed to treat chronic iron overload caused by frequent blood transfusions.

Similar to deferoxamine, their main purpose is to address iron overload rather than general heavy metal detoxification.

Possible side effects may include gastrointestinal disturbances, liver enzyme changes, and neutropenia (low white blood cell count).

Synthetic chelators are highly effective in addressing heavy metal poisoning. They serve as valuable tools, each designed for specific purposes, operating through distinct mechanisms, and carrying potential side effects. It is crucial to have thorough medical supervision and personalized treatment plans in order to optimize the advantages and minimize any potential risks.

CHAPTER THREE

Natural Chelators

Alpha Lipoic Acid

Natural chelators, such as alpha lipoic acid, are substances that can bind to and remove heavy metals and other toxins from the body. Alpha lipoic acid is a powerful antioxidant that can help protect against oxidative stress and support overall health.

Alpha Lipoic Acid (ALA) is an endogenous chemical present in all cells of the body. It serves as a potent antioxidant and possesses the exceptional capability to operate in both aqueous and lipid environments, rendering it extremely adaptable in the detoxification of different tissues.

ALA interacts with heavy metals such as mercury, arsenic, and lead, creating complexes that can be eliminated from the body. In addition, ALA stimulates the production of additional antioxidants, such as glutathione, so increasing the body's ability to eliminate toxins.

Applications:

- Heavy Metal Detoxification: Alpha-lipoic acid (ALA) is highly efficient in removing mercury and arsenic from the body through a process called chelation.

- Neurological Protection: ALA's capacity to penetrate the blood-brain barrier allows it to offer neuroprotective benefits, rendering it valuable in cases of mercury-induced neurotoxicity.

- Antioxidant: ALA provides general support for antioxidants by aiding in the regeneration of other antioxidants, hence promoting overall health and lowering oxidative stress.

Administration:

ALA can be taken orally as a supplement in the form of capsules or tablets. Trace amounts of it can also be found in foods such as spinach, broccoli, and potatoes.

Side Effects: ALA is generally well-tolerated, with few occurrences of side effects that are typically moderate in nature. Possible side effects of these medications include encompass gastrointestinal discomfort, skin irritations, and, when taken in excessive amounts, low blood sugar levels in individuals with diabetes.

Cilantro and Chlorella

Cilantro (Coriandrum sativum) and chlorella are commonly employed as natural chelators, which work in tandem to enhance the detoxification of heavy metals from the body. Cilantro can help remove heavy metals from the body's tissues and aid in their elimination. Its remarkable feature lies in its capacity to traverse the blood-brain barrier, facilitating the extraction of metals from the brain.

Chlorella, a variety of green algae, has the ability to attach to heavy metals in the intestines, therefore limiting their absorption and facilitating their elimination. Additionally, it contains a substantial amount of chlorophyll, which facilitates the process of detoxifying.

Uses:

- Mercury detoxification is commonly achieved by combining cilantro with chlorella, especially for the purpose of removing mercury from dental amalgams.

- General Detoxification: Both substances are employed in treatment plans aimed at diminishing the general accumulation of toxic heavy metals in the body, such as lead and aluminum.

Administration: Cilantro can be ingested in its raw state, as an extract, or in the form of a dietary supplement. Chlorella is commonly consumed in the form of a powder, pill, or capsule.

Adverse Reactions:

Cilantro: Adverse effects are infrequent but may encompass gastrointestinal disturbance and allergy responses.

Chlorella may cause gastrointestinal difficulties and, in certain instances, allergic responses as side effects. It is advisable to introduce Chlorella gradually in order to reduce any negative effects.

Garlic and other food-based chelators

Garlic:

Garlic (Allium sativum) is widely recognized for its several health advantages, including as its capacity to attach to and eliminate toxic heavy metals.

Mode of Operation: Garlic's sulfur-containing components, such allicin, attach to heavy metals such as lead and mercury, making it easier for the body to eliminate them.

Applications: Garlic is utilized for the purpose of eliminating lead, mercury, and cadmium toxins from the body, as well as promoting cardiovascular and immune system well-being.

Administration: Fresh garlic, garlic extracts, and supplements are frequently utilized. Ingesting raw garlic or aged garlic extract is especially advantageous.

Adverse Reactions: Adverse reactions may encompass gastrointestinal discomfort, halitosis, and, at elevated dosages, possible anticoagulant consequences.

Additional chelators derived from food sources:

Coriander

Coriander seeds has chelating capabilities similar to cilantro, which means they can aid in the mobilization of heavy metals.

Pectin

Pectin, which is present in apples and citrus fruits, has the ability to bind to heavy metals in the intestines, facilitating their elimination.

Turmeric

Turmeric contains curcumin, an active compound that has been proven to possess metal-binding capabilities and promotes liver detoxification.

Green Tea

Green tea, abundant in polyphenols, has the ability to increase the body's innate detoxifying mechanisms.

Herbal Chelation Remedies

- Milk Thistle (Silybum marianum):

Milk thistle is well-known for its hepatoprotective effects and aids in detoxification. The active component silymarin facilitates the regeneration of liver cells and promotes the formation of glutathione, hence assisting in the detoxification of heavy metals. Milk thistle is employed to promote liver well-being and facilitate the elimination of diverse poisons, such as heavy metals.

Milk thistle can be obtained in the form of a supplement, tincture, or tea. Generally well-tolerated, although it may induce minor stomach discomfort in certain individuals.

- Dandelion (Taraxacum officinale):

Dandelion root is routinely employed to promote liver and kidney functionality. It promotes the synthesis of bile and improves the liver's ability to remove toxins, facilitating the elimination of heavy metals.

Dandelion is utilized for the purpose of overall cleansing and to promote the well-being of the liver and kidneys. Dandelion root can be ingested in the form of a tea, tincture, or dietary supplement.

Adverse Reactions: Certain individuals may experience mild stomach pain.

- Burdock Root (Arctium lappa):

Burdock root is renowned for its ability to cleanse the blood. It facilitates the excretion of toxins via the skin and urine, promoting comprehensive detoxification.

Burdock root is utilized for the purpose of eliminating heavy metals from the body and promoting the well-being of the liver and kidneys. Burdock root can be consumed in the form of tea, tincture, or dietary supplement.

In general, most people can tolerate this medication well. However, a small number of individuals may develop allergic reactions or gastrointestinal discomfort.

Natural chelators offer a milder method for removing heavy metals from the body. Although natural chelators are generally safer and have fewer negative effects compared to synthetic chelators, their effectiveness and proper usage should be supervised by healthcare professionals, particularly in situations involving substantial exposure to heavy metals.

Protocols for Chelation Therapy

> ➢ Intravenous Chelation Therapy

Intravenous Chelation Therapy is a medical treatment that involves the administration of chelating agents through a vein. Intravenous (IV) chelation therapy is the process of delivering chelating chemicals directly into the bloodstream using an IV drip. This technique guarantees rapid and thorough assimilation of the chelating agent, rendering it exceptionally efficient for cases of acute and severe heavy metal poisoning.

Typical Agents Utilized:

- EDTA, also known as Ethylenediaminetetraacetic Acid, is frequently utilized for the purpose of lead and cardiovascular detoxification.

- DMPS (Dimercaptopropane-1-sulfonate) is the preferred substance for detoxifying mercury.

- Glutathione is occasionally employed in conjunction with chelators to enhance the process of detoxification and bolster antioxidant defense.

Method:

Initial Assessment: A comprehensive medical examination, which includes blood testing and a careful examination of medical records, to ascertain the specific type and degree of heavy metal exposure.

Preparation: The patient undergoes pre-treatment measures to ensure enough hydration and maintain a good balance of electrolytes before receiving IV therapy.

Administration: The chelating agent is administered intravenously at a slow rate, taking anywhere from 1 to 3 hours, depending on the specific protocol and the patient's condition.

Post-Therapy Monitoring: Patients undergo continuous monitoring for any negative responses throughout and following the infusion. Haematological and urinalysis examinations are performed to evaluate the efficacy of the treatment.

Advantages:

- Swift and efficient decrease in concentrations of heavy metals.
- By circumventing the digestive system, it guarantees full assimilation.
- Can be customized to suit specific requirements with accurate dosage.

Adverse Reactions:

- EDTA has the potential to cause hypocalcemia, which is characterized by low amounts of calcium.
- Potential renal strain necessitating meticulous monitoring of renal function.

- Common adverse reactions include mild symptoms such as tiredness, dizziness, and stomach discomfort.

CHAPTER FOUR

Oral Chelation Therapy

Oral chelation therapy refers to the administration of chelating chemicals through the mouth. This approach is more convenient and less intrusive compared to intravenous therapy, rendering it appropriate for prolonged detoxification and upkeep.

Common Agents Utilized:

DMSA (Dimercaptosuccinic Acid) is a highly effective substance for the detoxification of lead, mercury, and arsenic.

Alpha Lipoic Acid is a naturally occurring substance that acts as a chelator and has antioxidant characteristics.

Chlorella has the ability to attach to heavy metals in the digestive tract, facilitating their removal from the body.

Method:

Initial Assessment: Medical examination to ascertain the necessity for chelation therapy and select the proper dosage.

Dosing: The administration of the chelating agent is prescribed in precise amounts, typically consumed during meals to minimize pain in the gastrointestinal tract.

Monitoring: Regular scheduled appointments to observe progress and modify dosages as needed. Periodic blood and urine tests are performed.

Advantages:

- Efficient and unobtrusive.
- Appropriate for extended detoxification periods.
- Can be integrated with other detoxification treatments, such as modifications in diet.

Adverse Reactions:

- Gastrointestinal disturbances, such as feelings of nausea and episodes of diarrhea.
- Potential hypersensitivity responses to the chelating agent.
- Reduced bioavailability in comparison to intravenous delivery.

Methods of Chelation Administration

> Transdermal Chelation:

Involves the direct application of chelating chemicals to the skin. The chemicals penetrate the skin and enter the bloodstream. DMPS is frequently utilized in a topical formulation.

The chelating agent is administered into clean and dry skin, usually targeting areas with thin skin to enhance absorption. The application is executed in accordance with the prescribed process. This method is non-invasive and can be easily conducted in the comfort of one's own home.

Adverse Reactions: Possibility of skin irritation or allergic responses.

> Rectal chelation:

This process involves the rectal administration of chelating chemicals, which are then absorbed through the rectal mucosa. EDTA suppositories are commonly utilized.

The individual administers the suppository into the rectum, typically prior to going to sleep in order to facilitate absorption throughout the night.

Advantages: Circumvents the process of digestion, which may lead to a decrease in gastrointestinal adverse reactions.

Adverse Reactions:

Irritation or discomfort in the rectal area.

Utilizing a combination of chelation methods to achieve the most effective outcomes.

By utilizing a combination of chelation approaches, the process of detoxification can be optimized by targeting distinct areas of heavy metal accumulation, leading to improved overall health outcomes.

Approaches:

Sequential Utilization: Commencing with intravenous chelation for expeditious detoxification, succeeded by oral chelation for upkeep.

Simultaneous Use: The concurrent utilization of several chelation strategies, such as the simultaneous use of oral chelators in conjunction with dietary and lifestyle changes.

Supportive Therapies: Incorporating additional supportive therapies, such as antioxidant supplementation (e.g., vitamin C, glutathione), liver support (e.g., milk thistle), and dietary adjustments to increase the body's innate detoxification mechanisms.

Method:

Customized Strategy: An individualized treatment plan is created taking into account the patient's unique requirements, current health condition, and exposure to heavy metals.

Monitoring and Adjustments: Consistent surveillance using blood and urine tests to monitor advancement and modify regimens as needed.

Comprehensive Approach: Integrating modifications in lifestyle, dietary assistance, and additional complementary therapies to enhance overall well-being and the process of detoxification.

Advantages:

- Improved effectiveness of heavy metal detoxification.

- Minimized likelihood of adverse reactions by employing well-balanced and tailored methodologies.

- Enhanced overall physical and mental health and well-being.

Adverse Reactions:

- This therapy methods have become more sophisticated, necessitating meticulous coordination and monitoring.

- There is a possibility of interactions occurring between various chelating agents and supplements, which requires supervision from a specialist.

Chelation therapy procedures differ in terms of their approach, delivery, and efficacy. The most prevalent forms of chelation therapy are administered either intravenously or orally, each offering unique benefits and constraints. Topical and rectal administration methods offer alternate possibilities for individuals who are unable to tolerate conventional routes. By integrating various techniques and complementary treatments, one can enhance the effectiveness of detoxification, leading to a holistic approach in eliminating heavy metals and promoting overall well-being.

Applications and Benefits of Chelation Therapy

➢ Cardiovascular Health

Chelation therapy, first designed to address heavy metal intoxication, has been investigated for its potential advantages in cardiovascular health, namely in the management of atherosclerosis and associated heart conditions. EDTA (Ethylenediaminetetraacetic Acid) is the main substance employed in this situation. It has the ability to attach to metal ions and eliminate them from the body.

Mode of Operation

- **Atherosclerosis and Calcium Deposits:**

Atherosclerosis is characterized by the accumulation of plaques in the arteries, composed of lipids, cholesterol, calcium, and other compounds. These plaques have the ability to undergo calcification and stenosis of the arteries, so impeding blood circulation and resulting in cardiovascular conditions such coronary artery disease, myocardial infarctions, and cerebrovascular accidents.

- **EDTA Chelation:**

EDTA chelation involves the process of EDTA binding to both divalent and trivalent metal ions, such as calcium, which is a major constituent of atherosclerotic plaques. EDTA is believed to aid in the reduction of arterial plaque calcification by chelating and eliminating calcium from the bloodstream. This process has the potential to enhance arterial flexibility and improve blood flow.

Therapeutic Procedure:

- **Chelation Infusions:**

Patients usually undergo a sequence of 30 to 40 intravenous infusions of EDTA chelation solution. The duration of each session is around 3 to 4 hours, and it is conducted once or twice a week.

- **Adjunctive Therapy**

Adjunctive therapy involves the administration of supplementary supplements and drugs to enhance cardiovascular health. These may include antioxidants (such as vitamin

C), B-vitamins, magnesium, and heparin (to prevent the formation of blood clots).

It is crucial to regularly evaluate renal function, blood calcium levels, and cardiovascular health in order to guarantee safety and effectiveness.

Following the initial sequence of infusions, certain patients may undergo maintenance therapy, where they get recurrent chelation treatments to prolong the advantages.

Advantages

Decreased Cardiovascular Events: Chelation therapy has the potential to lower the likelihood of significant cardiovascular events, especially among high-risk groups such individuals with diabetes.

Enhanced Blood Flow: Chelation therapy has the ability to decrease arterial calcification and promote arterial flexibility, hence enhancing blood flow and the delivery of oxygen to the heart and other organs.

Potential hazards and adverse reactions

- Hypocalcemia can occur as a result of EDTA administration, which has the ability to decrease blood calcium levels. Common symptoms consist of muscle cramps, tingling sensations, and, in more severe instances, irregularities in heart rhythm known as cardiac arrhythmias.

- Kidney Strain: Chelation therapy can exacerbate the workload of the kidneys, especially in those with pre-existing renal problems. Consistent surveillance of renal function is essential.

- Gastrointestinal symptoms, such as nausea, vomiting, diarrhea, or abdominal discomfort, may be experienced by certain individuals during or after chelation infusions.

- Allergic responses to the chelating agent or other components of the infusion can occur, although they are uncommon.

Controversy and Criticism

- The application of chelation therapy for cardiovascular disease is still a subject of debate. While several researches demonstrate advantages, others have scrutinized the technique or discovered no substantial impacts.

- Medical Community Skepticism: Numerous cardiologists and mainstream medical organizations have a dubious stance towards chelation therapy for heart disease due to insufficient substantial proof and potential hazards.

- The regulatory status of chelation therapy is that it has been approved by the FDA for the treatment of heavy metal intoxication, but it has not been expressly approved for the treatment of cardiovascular disease. The off-label use of this medication for heart health should be explored with a healthcare provider.

Chelation therapy, namely using EDTA, exhibits potential as an adjunctive therapy for cardiovascular health by potentially diminishing arterial calcification and enhancing blood circulation. Nevertheless, the utilization of it is still a subject of debate and should be treated with prudence.

Individuals seeking chelation therapy for cardiovascular illness should seek guidance from their healthcare professional to carefully evaluate the potential advantages and drawbacks, and contemplate involvement in ongoing clinical trials to further examine its effectiveness and safety.

> **Neurological and Cognitive Health**

Alzheimer's Disease

Alzheimer's disease is a degenerative neurological ailment that progresses over time and is marked by a deterioration in cognitive function, loss of memory, and changes in behavior. Although the precise cause is uncertain, studies indicate that the development of the condition may be influenced by heavy metal poisoning.

Heavy metals and Alzheimer's disease:

Aluminum: Research has demonstrated that aluminum has the ability to build up in the brain, resulting in oxidative stress and neuroinflammation, both of which are significant characteristics of Alzheimer's disease. Aluminum has the potential to contribute to the development of beta-amyloid plaques, which are a characteristic feature of Alzheimer's disease.

Iron: An excessive amount of iron in the brain can accelerate the creation of reactive oxygen species, resulting in oxidative damage to neurons. Altered iron metabolism is evident in individuals with Alzheimer's disease.

Mercury: Prolonged exposure to mercury is linked to neurological harm, such as memory loss and cognitive impairment, which are indicative of Alzheimer's disease.

Chelation therapy for Alzheimer's disease:

EDTA Chelation:

The potential of EDTA to decrease aluminum and other heavy metal concentrations in the brain has been investigated. Preliminary studies indicate that chelation therapy may have a beneficial effect on reducing cognitive decline, although further research is required to confirm these findings.

Deferoxamine:

Deferoxamine, an iron chelator, has demonstrated potential in animal research and limited clinical trials. It has the potential to decrease the harmful effects of iron-induced oxidative damage in the brain and impede the advancement of Alzheimer's disease.

Obstacles and Factors to Take into Account:

The blood-brain barrier presents a hurdle in chelation therapy for Alzheimer's, as it hinders the direct removal of metals from brain tissue.

Clinical data: Although several trials show promise, there is currently a lack of robust clinical data to justify the regular use of chelation therapy for

Alzheimer's disease. Additional large-scale, randomized controlled trials are required.

> **Parkinson's Disease:**

Parkinson's disease is a neurodegenerative condition marked by the degeneration of dopaminergic neurons in the substantia nigra, resulting in motor symptoms as tremors, stiffness, and bradykinesia. Exposure to heavy metals is seen as a potential risk factor.

Heavy metals and Parkinson's disease:

- Manganese: Prolonged exposure to elevated levels of manganese is associated with manganism, a sickness similar to Parkinson's disease. Excessive amounts of manganese can harm dopaminergic neurons and lead to the development of symptoms associated with Parkinson's disease.

- Parkinson's patients often exhibit a common occurrence of iron buildup in the substantia nigra. An excessive amount of iron can worsen oxidative stress and cause damage to neurons.

- Copper: Abnormal copper metabolism may be a factor in the development of neurodegeneration in Parkinson's disease. Increased copper levels can facilitate the accumulation of alpha-synuclein, a protein implicated in the development of Parkinson's disease.

Chelation therapy for Parkinson's disease:

- Deferoxamine, an iron chelator, has been investigated for its ability to decrease iron buildup in the brain and alleviate neurodegeneration.

- Penicillamine, a substance that binds to copper, has been utilized in the treatment of Wilson's disease, a condition characterized by abnormal copper metabolism. It may also hold promise for those with Parkinson's disease who have elevated levels of copper.

For chelation therapy to be effective, it needs to specifically target and eliminate harmful metals while without disturbing the balance of necessary metals in the body.

Neuroprotective Strategies:

The combination of chelation therapy and antioxidant therapy may be necessary to optimize the advantages of neuroprotection.

> ➤ **Autism Spectrum Disorders.**

Autism Spectrum diseases (ASD) are a collection of neurodevelopmental diseases that are distinguished by difficulties in social communication and the presence of repetitive behaviors.

The etiology of ASD is complex, encompassing both genetic and environmental factors, which may include possible exposure to heavy metals.

Heavy metals and Autism Spectrum Disorder (ASD):

- Mercury: The exposure to mercury throughout pregnancy and early life has been associated with delays in neurodevelopment and impairments in cognitive function. Several studies indicate that children diagnosed with Autism Spectrum Disorder (ASD) may exhibit elevated amounts of mercury in their physiological systems.

- Lead exposure is linked to neurodevelopmental impairments, such as decreased IQ and difficulties with attention. Some children with ASD have been shown to have high levels of lead in their bodies.

- Aluminum: Aluminum exposure is linked to neurotoxicity, and several studies have examined its possible involvement in ASD, however the evidence remains equivocal.

Chelation therapy for Autism Spectrum Disorder (ASD):

Dimercaptosuccinic Acid (DMSA) is the most extensively researched chelator for Autism Spectrum Disorder (ASD). Several studies have documented enhancements in symptoms after chelation therapy with DMSA, although the findings are inconsistent and subject to debate.

EDTA, a chelating agent, has been used in certain circumstances to treat children with Autism Spectrum Disorder (ASD) despite lacking official approval. However, the effectiveness and safety of this treatment are still a subject of ongoing discussion and uncertainty.

Safety Concerns: Chelation therapy carries the risk of notable adverse effects, such as renal impairment, hypocalcemia, and gastrointestinal disruptions. The potential drawbacks may exceed the advantages in youngsters.

The medical community has conflicting opinions regarding the use of chelation therapy for ASD. Although a few practitioners claim beneficial results, professional medical organizations often do not support it because of limited proof and potential hazards.

Additional comprehensive and extensive research are required to assess the safety and effectiveness of chelation therapy for Autism Spectrum Disorder (ASD).

Chelation therapy exhibits promise in addressing health problems associated with heavy metal exposure in individuals with Alzheimer's, Parkinson's, and Autism Spectrum Disorders. However, its use is still a subject of controversy and should be addressed with prudence. Although initial research shows promise, additional rigorous clinical evidence is required to validate its effectiveness and safety. Patients contemplating chelation therapy should seek the assistance of a competent healthcare professional, who will closely monitor and assess the potential dangers and benefits.

> ### **Detoxification**

Improving Liver Function

The liver has a crucial function in the body's detoxification process, since it metabolizes and eliminates different pollutants, such as heavy metals. Optimizing liver function is crucial for the efficacy of chelation therapy, since it facilitates the body's capacity to metabolize and excrete chelated metals.

Dietary Support:

- Milk Thistle (Silybum marianum) is a plant that contains silymarin, a chemical renowned for its hepatoprotective and regenerative qualities. Silymarin promotes hepatic cell regeneration and elevates glutathione levels, a crucial antioxidant involved in liver detoxification.

- N-Acetyl Cysteine (NAC) is a compound that serves as a precursor to glutathione, an essential substance for the liver's detoxification functions. Supplementing with NAC enhances glutathione levels and promotes liver health.

- Turmeric, scientifically known as Curcuma longa, is a plant that contains a compound called curcumin. Curcumin is known for its ability to reduce inflammation and act as an antioxidant. Curcumin aids in the process of liver detoxification and safeguards liver cells against harm.

- Dandelion Root (Taraxacum officinale) is commonly employed for its hepatoprotective properties and its ability to facilitate liver function and detoxification. It stimulates the generation of bile and improves the liver's capacity to digest and eliminate pollutants.

Changes in lifestyle:

- Hydration: Proper hydration promotes liver function by aiding in the removal of toxins through urine.

- Nutrition: Consuming a diet abundant in fruits, vegetables, whole grains, and lean proteins supplies vital nutrients and antioxidants that promote the well-being of the liver.

- To limit the liver's detoxification workload, it is advisable to reduce exposure to alcohol, processed meals, and environmental pollutants.

Advantages

Enhanced detoxification: Improving liver function facilitates the more effective processing and removal of chelated metals, hence decreasing the likelihood of re-toxification.

Supporting liver function with chelation therapy can help reduce oxidative stress and inflammation, both of which are commonly increased in persons receiving this treatment.

General Well-being: A well-functioning liver enhances general physical condition, facilitates digestion, and boosts energy levels.

> **Enhancing Kidney Health**

The kidneys have a crucial function in the filtration of blood and the elimination of waste substances, such as chelated heavy metals. Ensuring optimal kidney function is essential during chelation therapy to facilitate the effective elimination of toxins from the body and to safeguard against renal impairment.

Hydration

Sufficient water consumption is crucial for preserving renal function and aiding in the elimination of chelated metals. It is advisable to have a minimum of 8-10 glasses of water daily.

Herbal Support:

Cranberry Extract is recognized for its capacity to promote urinary tract health and prevent infections, making it advantageous in the context of chelation therapy.

Nettle Leaf (Urtica dioica) functions as a diuretic, stimulating the production of urine and aiding in the elimination of harmful substances from the kidneys.

Dietary assistance:

Antioxidants such as Vitamins C and E, as well as selenium and zinc, aid in safeguarding kidney cells against oxidative harm during chelation therapy.

Magnesium aids in maintaining optimal kidney function and mitigates the likelihood of kidney stone development, a potential issue during chelation therapy.

Changes in lifestyle:

Minimizing the intake of nephrotoxic chemicals, such as nonsteroidal anti-inflammatory medications (NSAIDs) and specific antibiotics, is crucial to protect the kidneys.

Continuous Monitoring: Periodic blood and urine tests are conducted to closely monitor the functioning of the kidneys and identify any initial indications of renal stress or impairment.

Advantages

Optimal Toxin Removal: Ensuring kidney health facilitates the efficient filtration and excretion of chelated metals and other pollutants from the body.

Preventing kidney Damage: Implementing protective measures and conducting regular monitoring will help prevent any renal damage that may be related with chelation therapy.

General Health: Optimal kidney function plays a crucial role in maintaining overall well-being, ensuring appropriate equilibrium of fluids and electrolytes, as well as regulating blood pressure.

> **Immune System Benefits:**

Chelation therapy, through the reduction of heavy metal accumulation in the body, can yield substantial advantages for the immune system. Heavy metals have the ability to inhibit immunological function, which increases the vulnerability of the body to infections and chronic diseases. Boosting the immune system while undergoing chelation therapy improves overall well-being and aids the body in efficiently combating and recovering from heavy metal poisoning.

Dietary Assistance:

- Vitamin C is a powerful antioxidant that helps boost the immune system by shielding immune cells from oxidative harm and improving the synthesis and effectiveness of white blood cells.

- Zinc is crucial for the optimal functioning of the immune system since it plays a vital role in the formation and activation of immune cells. Additionally, it possesses antioxidant characteristics that safeguard against oxidative stress.

- Vitamin D is essential for regulating the immune response and boosting the ability of monocytes and macrophages to fight against pathogens.

- Probiotics promote gastrointestinal health, which is intricately connected to immune system function. An optimal gut microbiota contributes to the maintenance of a harmonized immune response.

Herbal Support:

Echinacea: Echinacea, renowned for its immunostimulatory characteristics, aids in the proliferation of leukocytes and augments the body's capacity to combat infections.

Astragalus: Astragalus is an adaptogenic herb that enhances immune function by boosting the activity of white blood cells and enhancing resilience to stress.

Implementing changes to one's lifestyle:

Sufficient sleep, typically 7-8 hours each night, is crucial for supporting the immune system since it enables the body to undergo repair and regeneration processes.

Engaging in regular exercise: Engaging in moderate physical activity improves the functioning of the immune system and aids in the reduction of inflammation.

Stress Management: Prolonged stress might inhibit the functioning of the immune system. Activities such as meditation, yoga, and deep breathing exercises aid in the management of stress and promote the health of the immune system.

Advantages

Enhance Immune Function: Chelation therapy can enhance immune function by lowering the accumulation of heavy metals and providing support to the immune system. This can result in improved resistance to infections and chronic diseases.

Diminished Inflammation: Heavy metals have the potential to contribute to the development of chronic inflammation, which is associated with a range of health problems. Chelation therapy aids in the reduction of inflammation and promotes general immune system well-being.

General Health and Well-Being: A robust immune system enhances general health, boosts energy levels, and enhances quality of life.

It is essential to enhance liver and kidney function, as well as boost the immune system, while undergoing chelation therapy in order to optimize its advantages and reduce potential hazards. Chelation therapy relies on nutritional assistance, herbal medicines, lifestyle modifications, and regular monitoring to ensure its effectiveness and safety. Through the enhancement of these crucial activities, persons who undergo chelation therapy can attain superior detoxification, enhanced health outcomes, and a more robust immune response.

CHAPTER FIVE

Diet, Lifestyle, and Chelation

Proper nutrition is essential for helping the detoxification process during chelation therapy. These dietary options can improve the effectiveness of chelation therapy and increase general health.

Antioxidant-Rich Foods: To prevent oxidative stress produced by heavy metals, eat foods high in antioxidants such as berries, leafy greens, and nuts.

Mineral Support: Make sure you're getting enough zinc, magnesium, and calcium, which can all be depleted during chelation. Foods high in these minerals include seeds, nuts, whole grains, and dairy.

Fiber-rich foods: Consume high-fiber foods, such as fruits, vegetables, and whole grains, to help heavy metals pass through the digestive system.

Hydration: Drink enough of water to help remove toxins from the body and maintain kidney function during detoxing.

Detoxifying Herbs and Supplements: The benefits of herbs and supplements including cilantro, chlorella, garlic, and spirulina, are believed to aid in detoxification process.

Lifestyle Practices to Improve Effective Chelation

In addition to dietary changes, some lifestyle activities can help to improve the effectiveness of chelation therapy and create a toxin-free body:

Exercise: Exercise on a regular basis to improve circulation, lymphatic system support, and toxin clearance through sweat.

Sauna Therapy: Use sauna sessions to increase sweating and aid in the removal of toxins from the body. Infrared saunas are especially useful for detoxification.

Stress Management: Stress-reduction practices such as meditation, yoga, and deep breathing exercises can help you feel better and lower the strain on your body's detoxification processes.

Sleep hygiene: Maintain ample and restful sleep to help the body's natural detoxification processes and general wellness.

Avoiding Toxins: Reduce your exposure to environmental pollutants by using natural cleaning products, avoiding processed foods, and purchasing organic produce wherever feasible.

Avoiding Re-exposure to heavy metals

Preventing re-exposure to heavy metals is critical for extending the advantages of chelation therapy and protecting your health. These are practical suggestions for lowering your risk of heavy metal exposure:

Water Quality: Use a high-quality water filter to ensure that your drinking water is free of impurities such as heavy metals and poisons.

Dietary Choices: Be careful of the origins of your food, avoiding mercury-rich fish and seafood, and choosing organic products to prevent pesticide exposure.

Household Products: Use non-toxic household products such as natural cleaning supplies, heavy metal-free cookware, and chemical-free personal care products.

Workplace Safety: If you operate in an environment where you may be exposed to heavy metals, observe safety requirements, wear protective equipment, and ensure enough ventilation.

Environmental Awareness: Stay aware about local environmental risks and take efforts to decrease your exposure, such as avoiding high-pollution areas and utilizing air purifiers at home.

Combining nutritional assistance, lifestyle behaviors, and proactive efforts to minimize re-exposure will help you maximize the advantages of chelation therapy and support your road to optimal health. This holistic approach keeps your body toxin-free and vibrant, allowing you to reap the full benefits of chelation therapy for years to come.

Ensuring Safety and Managing Risk

Understanding Potential Risks

While chelation therapy has many health benefits, it is important to be informed of the potential hazards and consequences of the treatment.

Nutrient Depletion: Chelation agents can bind to important minerals including calcium, magnesium, and zinc, causing shortages. Understanding and managing this risk is critical for overall health.

Kidney and Liver Stress: The process of excreting heavy metals can put additional strain on the kidneys and liver, particularly in people with preexisting problems.

Allergic Reactions: Some people may have allergic reactions to chelating drugs, which can vary from minor skin rashes to severe anaphylaxis.

Hypocalcemia: Rapid calcium removal can result in hypocalcemia, a disorder marked by low calcium levels in the blood that can induce muscle cramps, spasms, and heart problems.

Managing Side Effects

Common side effects of chelation therapy include nausea, vomiting, diarrhea, and stomach discomfort. Side effects must be managed properly to ensure a safe and effective chelation therapy experience. These are the ways for minimizing and managing common side effects.

- Supplementation: Monitor and supply critical nutrients that may be depleted during chelation therapy, such as calcium, magnesium, zinc, and other minerals.

- Maintain enough water to promote renal function and aid in the removal of chelated metals.

- Gradual Dosage Adjustments: Begin with minimal doses of chelating drugs and gradually increase to reduce side effects and allow the body to adjust.

- Monitoring & Testing: Regular blood tests should be performed to check electrolyte levels, renal function, and liver health. Adjust treatment regimens in response to test results to guarantee safety.

- Symptom Management: Use pharmaceuticals or natural therapies to treat nausea, gastrointestinal pain, and allergic responses. Consult a healthcare professional for specific guidance.

- Rest and recovery: Allow enough time between treatment sessions for the body to repair and adapt to the detoxification process.

Ensuring Safe and Effective Treatment

To maximize the benefits of chelation therapy while avoiding hazards, it is critical to follow safe and effective treatment protocols.

- Seek treatment from competent and trained healthcare providers who specialize in chelation therapy. Check their credentials and track record to confirm competence.

- Before beginning chelation therapy, conduct a comprehensive health examination to detect any contraindications or prior diseases that may necessitate specific precautions.

- Work with your healthcare practitioner to create a personalized treatment plan based on your unique needs, health status, and goals.

- Regular Monitoring: Schedule regular follow-up appointments to track progress, adapt treatment procedures, and swiftly address any emergent difficulties.

- Informed Consent: Make sure you understand the risks, benefits, and alternatives to chelation therapy. Give informed permission based on a thorough comprehension of the treatment procedure.

- Emergency Preparedness: Be prepared for potential crises by having access to emergency medical care and understanding the symptoms of severe adverse reactions that necessitate quick attention.

-

By knowing potential dangers, effectively controlling side effects, and maintaining safe treatment methods, you can improve the outcomes of chelation therapy and your overall health and well-being. This complete approach prepares you to make informed decisions and boldly traverse the path to detoxification and good health.

Advancements in Chelation Delivery Methods

Chelation therapy delivery technologies have advanced, making treatments more effective, accessible, and patient-friendly.

Oral Chelation: Advancements in oral chelation formulations that improve absorption and bioavailability, offering a more practical alternative to intravenous therapy.

Transdermal Chelation: The creation of transdermal patches and creams that enable chelating chemicals to be absorbed via the skin, providing a non-invasive delivery technique.

Sustained-Release Formulations: The introduction of chelation treatments with controlled, progressive chelating agent release, which improves patient compliance and reduces side effects.

Nanotechnology: The use of nanotechnology to create chelating agents contained in nanoparticles, which improve their capacity to pass biological barriers and reach specific regions.

Integrating Chelation with Other Therapies

When combined with other therapeutic methods, chelation therapy can be an effective component of a comprehensive treatment approach. This following investigates the synergistic effects of combining chelation and other treatments:

- Nutritional Therapy: Nutritional therapy combines chelation with personalized nutritional regimens to replace depleted nutrients, promote detoxification pathways, and improve general health.

- Herbal Medicine: Using herbal supplements with detoxifying and supporting characteristics, such as milk thistle, dandelion root, and turmeric, to supplement chelation therapy.

- Hyperbaric Oxygen Therapy (HBOT): HBOT is used to improve chelation effectiveness by increasing oxygenation, decreasing inflammation, and promoting tissue healing.

- Intravenous Vitamin Therapy: The use of intravenous vitamins and minerals in conjunction with chelation to offer immediate replenishment of key nutrients while also supporting the detoxification process.

- Physical Therapies: Physical therapies include massage, acupuncture, and chiropractic care to enhance circulation, relieve stress, and aid the body's natural detoxification processes.

- Lifestyle modifications: Making lifestyle modifications such as stress management strategies, exercise routines, and avoiding environmental toxins in order to maximize the advantages of chelation therapy and improve long-term health.

END

www.ingramcontent.com/pod-product-compliance
Lightning Source LLC
Chambersburg PA
CBHW071936210526
45479CB00002B/703